YOUR KNOWLEDGE HAS VALUE

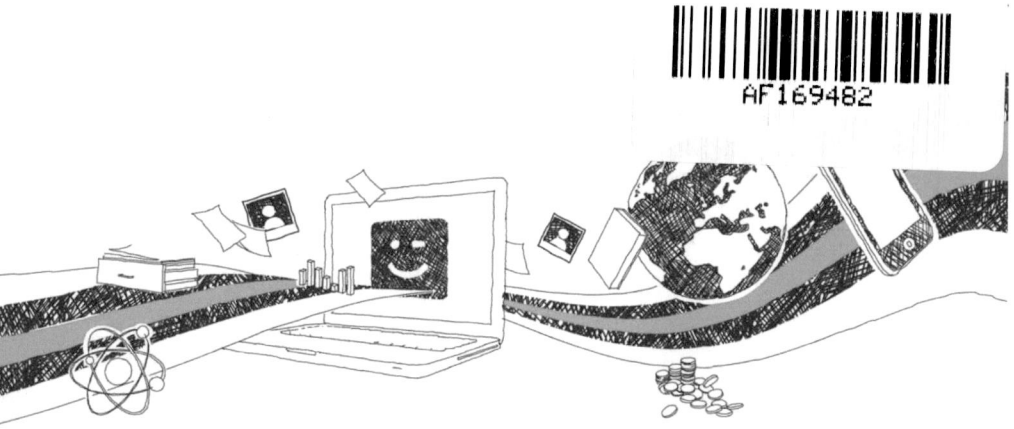

- We will publish your bachelor's and master's thesis, essays and papers

- Your own eBook and book - sold worldwide in all relevant shops

- Earn money with each sale

Upload your text at www.GRIN.com
and publish for free

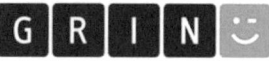

Bibliographic information published by the German National Library:

The German National Library lists this publication in the National Bibliography; detailed bibliographic data are available on the Internet at http://dnb.dnb.de .

This book is copyright material and must not be copied, reproduced, transferred, distributed, leased, licensed or publicly performed or used in any way except as specifically permitted in writing by the publishers, as allowed under the terms and conditions under which it was purchased or as strictly permitted by applicable copyright law. Any unauthorized distribution or use of this text may be a direct infringement of the author s and publisher s rights and those responsible may be liable in law accordingly.

Imprint:

Copyright © 2014 GRIN Verlag, Open Publishing GmbH
Print and binding: Books on Demand GmbH, Norderstedt Germany
ISBN: 9783668297074

This book at GRIN:

http://www.grin.com/en/e-book/339919/novel-drug-delivery-systems-for-the-delivery-of-insulin

Radhika Narain

Novel drug delivery systems for the delivery of Insulin

GRIN Publishing

GRIN - Your knowledge has value

Since its foundation in 1998, GRIN has specialized in publishing academic texts by students, college teachers and other academics as e-book and printed book. The website www.grin.com is an ideal platform for presenting term papers, final papers, scientific essays, dissertations and specialist books.

Visit us on the internet:

http://www.grin.com/

http://www.facebook.com/grincom

http://www.twitter.com/grin_com

A Review Article
NOVEL DRUG DELIVERY SYSTEMS FOR THE DELIVERY OF INSULIN

ABSTRACT

The delivery of proteins is challenging due to their high molecular weight and hydrophilic structures, making them difficult to cross the ubiquitous lipidic membranes. Proteins have a unique structure which makes them suited to a unique function, therefore, maintenance of the structural integrity and stability of these macromolecules is also of a high concern as they can easily be denatured by temperature, pH and other physiochemical changes. The protein and peptide delivery systems have to be designed in a way such that the drug carriers can protect the protein from proteases, increase its permeability through membranes, increase its absorption and bioavailability, sustain its release, with low dosage requirements and, increase its systemic circulation. The study presents the delivery of insulin through various routes: buccal, transdermal, oral and pulmonary, utilizing different novel carriers like polymeric nanoparticles, solid lipid nanoparticles, liposomes, nanoshells, nanospheres and nanoparticles encapsulated in microparticles, along with drug surface modification either by attaching peptide ligands or conjugating with polymers to enhance absorption and targeting capacity of the drug.

Key Words: peptides, insulin, oral, transdermal, buccal, pulmonary

INTRODUCTION

The biological nanomolecules or "nanomotors" inside the body like proteins and nucleic acids play a drastic role in determining the activity or behavior of organisms every second so that homeostasis is maintained. An imbalance in even a single process at the transcriptional, translational and/or post-translational level can lead to a misbalance or a diseased state. The healing process can be designed by utilizing these biological substances to influence the body more naturally. Drug delivery scientists have made only a few attempts towards the improvement of human health using biological substances, in contrast to artificially synthesized drugs, for delivery *in vivo* or *in vitro*. The conventional delivery systems to deliver these therapeutics face certain challenges, leading to the birth of novel drug delivery systems.

Challenges faced by conventional drug delivery systems: The conventional drug delivery systems suffer from many drawbacks such as poor stability, low systemic bioavalability, low drug solubility and absorption, rapid first pass metabolism, frequent and large dosing, uncontrolled release, lower drug targeting, lower cellular and intracellular uptake, and reduced drug half-life . The traditional invasive delivery techniques lead to a poor patient compliance and combined with the above shortcomings, the conventional delivery system may lead to the overall failure of treatment.

Novel drug delivery systems: The abovementioned problems faced by the conventional delivery systems can be solved by novel drug delivery systems which mainly entail the use of nanoparticulate drug delivery systems (NPDDS). The nanoparticles are particles in the range of 1-100 nm which can be divided into inorganic, polymeric or solid lipid nanoparticles. They are able to solve the problems created by the conventional drug delivery systems by controlling drug release, increasing drug permeability, solubility and bioavalability, especially for hydrophilic drugs. The drug loading, stability and encapsulation efficiency can be enhanced using NPDDS and the drug can be delivered through various routes including oral, buccal, pulmonary, parenteral, transdermal, ocular and brain. Moreover, the nanoparticles can be manipulated to enhance permeation and achieve targeting by surface functionalizing or attaching site-specific ligands like polyethylene glycol (PEG). They can also be made "smart" by making them stimuli responsive internally (sensitive to pH, temperature or light) and externally (sensitive to magnetic and electric fields).

Delivery of proteins and peptides: A peptide is a polymeric sequence of amino acids up to 50 monomers but if the number of amino acids exceeds 50, the polymer is generally described as a protein, which can assume the tertiary and quaternary configuration. The structure of the protein determines its function. Therefore, it is imperative that the protein maintains its structure before reaching the target where it can bring about its required function. Chemical and physical stability of the protein drug is essential for the proper function of the protein. The stability is intrinsically dependent on the primary, secondary, tertiary and quaternary structure of proteins, and extrinsically on the pH, temperature, moisture, concentration and excipients.

Looking at the chemistry, amino acids have different functional groups. They may take part in reactions like deamidation, oxidation, disulfide bridging leading to chemical degradation. They may also decide the non-polar and polar character of the peptide or provide a wide range of pK_a values determining physical characteristics like solubility or transport through aqueous media or lipidic membranes inside the body. The functional groups alone are responsible for the function of peptides since they can only form primary or secondary structures. The function of the proteins, on the other hand, is dependent on the maintenance of the exact 3-D structure.

Protein unfolding/denaturation and aggregation are two important challenges faced in drug delivery. If unfolding takes place, the structure and hence, the function of the protein will be affected. Folding of the protein in aqueous media occurs so that the protein acquires the thermodynamically stable state, whereby it hides its non-polar residues by hydrophobic interactions. More folding may be brought about by hydrogen bonding, van der Waals interactions and cystinal disulfide bridges. Unfolding may occur due to alteration in pH, temperature or ionic strength. It may be reversible upon reverting the conditions to the original, or irreversible (as in aggregation) wherein partial unfolding followed by re-folding changes the protein structure and hence, its function. Thus, gastric pH environment and proteases are impediments for protein delivery through oral route[i]. Aggregation also makes the protein inactive due to lumping of individual protein molecules together. It also makes it difficult for proteins to be suspended in solution, leading to precipitation. Proteins may also adsorb on various interfaces as they possess an active surface.

Moreover, proteins, unlike other small drugs, are high molecular weight cumbersome "macro" molecules which cannot cross the tight junctions in the epithelium. The proteins and peptides are hydrophilic molecules which face the basic problem of transport across lipophilic cell membrane barriers. This problem has been overcome by the emergent cell penetrating peptides (CPPs) or Trojan peptides as they can carry the attached cargo across the plasma membrane into the cell[ii]. Tingting Fan et al . designed peptide ligand modified SLNs (sCT-CSK-SLNs and sCT-IRQ-SLNs) to deliver salmon calcitonin (sCT) orally, using IRQRRRR (IRQ) as a CPP and CSKSSDYQC (CSK) as a goblet cell targeting peptide. The carriers were shown to improve drug internalization on Caco-2/HT29-MTX co-cultured cells via clathrin and caveolae dependent endocytosis and increased drug bioavailability to $12.41 \pm 3.65\%$ (sCT CSK-SLNs) and $10.05 \pm 5.10\%$ (sCT IRQ-SLNs) compared with $5.07 \pm 0.54\%$ (unmodified SLNs), when administered intraduodenally to rats[iii].

The most common route of protein delivery is the parental route, which includes subcutaneous, intravenous and intramuscular injections, but entails poor patient compliance. There are various other routes of delivery which involve non-invasive delivery techniques. The pulmonary route has the advantage of a highly vascularized network in the lungs with a large surface area that favors absorption through inhalation (non-invasive delivery). The nasal cavity is also extensively vascularized and the nasal tissue highly permeable, with low proteolytic activity and avoidance of liver first pass effect. The olfactory region can be targeted through which the drug passes directly into the brain. However, both the pulmonary and nasal routes have rapid mucociliary clearance, which is a limiting factor. The transdermal route can be utilized with techniques like sonoporation, iontophoresis, electroporation etc. to increase the permeation through the stratum corneum of the skin. The ocular delivery route has to overcome the following barriers to become successful: poor corneal permeability, blurred vision, nasolacrimal drainage, systemic absorption, tear turnover, poor drainage of instilled solutions[iv]. Due to these factors, it is not a preferred route for systemic delivery of proteins; it has only been used for local ocular disorders. The delivery of proteins and peptides to the brain is hampered by the blood brain barrier (BBB). Peptides serving as neuropeptides have immense potential to serve as therapeutic agents targeting the brain. The oral route has been most widely studied but presents problems such as gastric pH instability, high protease content in the upper gastrointestinal tract, the epithelial and mucosa barrier.

In the present study, the delivery of insulin has been presented in detail, casting light upon different delivery routes, their advantages and disadvantages and recent works.

DELIVERY OF INSULIN

The discovery of insulin, a polypeptide hormone secreted from the pancreatic β cells of islets of langerhans, as a therapeutic drug has been a turning point in drug discovery. Since the development of the first genetically produced human insulin in 1982, more than 200 genetically produced proteins and peptides have been developed to serve as human therapeutics[ii].

Insulin has the following noteworthy properties influencing its biological and therapeutic activity:
- It has a hydrophobic centre due to the energetically favourable alignment of uncharged amino acids inside, and a hydrophilic outer surface due to the presence of charged amino acids outside, making it unable to cross the lipidic membrane barriers.
- It is a macromolecule and thus, it cannot pass through the tightly packed biological membranes, as in the case of the tight junctions of epithelium.

It is used for the treatment of insulin dependent type I diabetes (diabetes mellitus) and many non-insulin dependent type II diabetes. The treatment entails long term therapies with insulin pumps and subcutaneous (s.c.) injections as the commonly used treatments. The daily multiple s.c. injections are considered as the standard treatments by diabetics[v] but they present a number of disadvantages: injection pain, poor patience compliance, risk of infection and transmission of diseases, expensive due to daily injections and frequent visits to the hospital, hypertrophy (enlargement of cells around injection site) and lypodystrophy (loss of fat at injection site), micro- and macroangiopathy, insulin oedema and atherosclerosis[vi]. Non-insulin dependent patients may develop 'psychological insulin resistance' or needle anxiety[vii,viii].

The goal of introduction of exogenous insulin in diabetics is to mimic the normal insulin activity in non-diabetics[ix] but s.c. injections fail to mimic it as all tissues are exposed to an equal insulin concentration, leaving the liver with only 20% of initially injected insulin, which has negative effects like hypertrophy[x]. Moreover, s.c. injected insulin bypasses the liver 1st pass effect in contrast to normal insulin pharmacodynamic profile leading to higher insulin exposure to tissues (hyperinsulaemic effects)[ix]. Therefore, other delivery routes have been explored, having their own advantages and shortcomings.

Oral delivery: The oral route for insulin delivery has been most widely and extensively studied as it overcomes the drawbacks from invasive delivery techniques like s.c. injections. However, it faces some impediments like gastric pH instability in the stomach, proteolytic enzyme content in the upper GI tract, low permeability across intestinal epithelial cells (paracelullar transport through tight junctions) and mucus layer, and first-pass metabolism in the liver. These factors affect the bioavailability, stability and integrity of insulin delivered through the oral route and have to be overcome while preparing an oral formulation of insulin.

Polymer based nanoparticles (NPs), gold nanoparticles, liposomes and solid lipid nanoparticles (SLNs) have been used with drug or carrier modifications (conjugation with peptide ligands or polymers), to deliver insulin orally. Pedro Fonte et al. (2015) extensively reviewed both synthetic and natural polymer based NPs for oral insulin delivery, concluding that dextran sulfate complexed with chitosan NPs were able to retain insulin in acidic medium of the stomach; alginate/chitosan NPs could encapsulate insulin with a high drug loading (14.3%) and were able to preserve the secondary structure of insulin; hyaluronic acid NPs increased insulin uptake through the intestine; versatile NPs could be made with PLGA since it could be combined with other polymers and coated with different ligands like cationic chitosan, PEGlyation and functionalizing with cell penetrating peptides (CPPs) could be further done to improve bioavailability; PCL NPs had a slower degradation than PLGA NPs, and; acrylic polymer NPs could inhibit proteolytic activity, alter cell tight junctions and enhance mucoadhesion. Since, biodegradable polymeric NPs present toxicology concerns like accumulation inside cells, they are not in use[xi].

Xingwang Zhang et al. (2014) developed biotinylated liposomes (BLPs) to enhance oral bioavalability of insulin as compared to conventional liposomes (CLPs). On oral administration to diabetic rats, the relative pharmacological bioavailability was 12.09% and 6.36% for the BLPs and CLPs, respectively. C_{max} in plasma for insulin loaded BLPs (20 IU/kg) was 52 µIU/mL and for insulin loaded CLPs (20 IU/kg) was 16 µIU/mL at a T_{max} of 5 hours whereas, for insulin solution (s.c., 1 IU/kg), it was 122 µIU/mL at a T_{max} of 45 minutes, showing the mild efficacy of BLPs and prolonged therapeutic affect (phamacological activity of BLPs lasted for 12 h in contrast to 5 h for s.c. insulin solution)[xii].

Xiang Yuan Xiong et al. (2013) developed pluronic P85/poly(lactic acid) vesicles showing that insulin loaded polymer vesicles had a gradual parabolic release profile spread within 8 hours (74% and 96% insulin release at 2.5 and 7.5 hours, respectively) in contrast to free insulin which had a more abrupt release profile spread within 2.5 hours (100% insulin release at 2.5 hours)[xiii].

Xiuying Li et al. (2013) used core shell corona nanolipoparticles (CSC) ('core' = chitosan NPs (NC); 'shell' = pluronic F127-lipid vesicles, and; 'corona' = polyethylene oxide) to ameliorate the absorption and bioavailability of insulin and to protect insulin from enzymatic degradation and showed that the amount of insulin permeated across rat ileum from NC was approximately 6, 14, 26, 35 ng and from CSC was approximately 10, 21, 44, 62 ng in 0.5, 1, 1.5, 2 hours, respectively, showing a higher permeation for insulin in CSC than in NC in the same time. The enzyme degradation studies showed that in presence of trypsin, free insulin degraded completely in 1 hour whereas, only 58% insulin from CSC degraded at the same time. In the presence of chymotrypsin, 92% of the free insulin and 42% of insulin from CSC degraded in 2 hours, showing the higher enzymatic resistance of the CSC insulin[xiv]. Piyasi Mukopadhyay et al. (2015) conducted a similar study using chitosan/alginate core-shell NPs showing that relative bioavailability of insulin along with the carrier was approximately 8.11%[xv].

Hyun-Jong Cho et al. (2014) synthesized chondroitin sulfate (CS)-capped gold NPs loaded with insulin (AuNPs/INS) and showed that glucose levels in diabetic rats went down by 32% in 1 hour for AuNPs/INS compared to the basal insulin level in rats. The insulin concentration in plasma at 2 hours after administration was 0.36 ± 0.30 μU/mL and 2.38 ± 1.52 μU/mL for free insulin solution and AuNPs/INS, respectively[xvi].

Fei Yu et al. (2015) constructed INS-loaded polymer–lipid hybrid nanoparticles (INS-PLGA-lipid-PEG NPs) followed by formulation of the spherical micro-particles using a spray freeze dryer (SFD), with a microfluidic aerosol nozzle (MFAN), forming uniform particles (212 μm) to improve the delivery efficiency of insulin. The pharmacodynamic study revealed that the blood glucose level in diabetic rats after oral administration declined by almost 10% and 50%

in 10 hours for oral enteric-coated capsule filled with the microparticles containing INS-PLGA-lipid-PEG NPs (40 IU/kg) and s.c. injection of the free INS (51 IU/kg), respectively[xvii].

Buccal delivery: Buccal delivery is a form of oral delivery which has the same advantages as that oral delivery system but at the same time avoids its shortcomings. It evades the acidic environment of the GI tract and has comparatively low enzyme content as compared to the oral delivery route. It bypasses the hepatic first-pass metabolism, directly entering the systemic circulation and also saves insulin against the presystemic metabolism, leading to higher insulin bioavailability[xviii-xxi]. In addition, it is highly vascularized, offering a good amount of surface area for insulin absorption[xxii]. Buccal epithelium is devoid of a keratinized layer, adding on to its advantages. However, the mucosal barrier properties remain intact and the constant flow of saliva causes dilution or decrease in the drug concentration[xxiii]. Also, the buccal barrier is multilayered. Due to this reason, mucoadhesive polymers are utilized as drug carriers.

J. O. Morales et al. (2014) prepared insulin coated nanopaticles (ICNPs) embedded in polymeric films of polymethacrylate derivative (ERL) or a combination of ERL with hydroxypropyl methylcellulose (HPMC) and showed that the cumulative permeated insulin through *in vitro* tridimensional human buccal mucosa model was approximately 53% (ICNPs+ERL), 8% (ICNPs+ERL+HPMC) and 0% (pure valine NPs w/o insulin; control) in 4 hours. Mucus diffusion study showed that P_{app} of sCT CSK-SLNs and sCT IRQ-SLNs was $4.05 \pm 0.43 \times 10^{-5}$ cm/s and $4.52 \pm 0.41 \times 10^{-5}$ cm/s, respectively as compared to that of unmodified SLNs ($2.79 \pm 0.34 \times 10^{-5}$ cm/s, proving that the mucus had an important role on the transport of SLNs, particularly unmodified ones[xxiv].

Concetta Giovino et al. (2012) developed insulin loaded polymeric NPs (made of poly(ethylene glycol)methyl ether-block-polylactide (PEG-b-PLA)) and embedded them in mucoadhesive chitosan films. The *in vitro* insulin release profile with a dialysis membrane in PBS at a pH of 6.8 and 37°C, (mimicking human buccal physiological conditions) from these insulin loaded carriers showed a biphasic sustained release over 35 days controlled by pH of media. In the first phase, 40% of insulin was released in 6 hours (due to burst effect of adsorbed insulin on NP surface) followed by the sustained release profile in the second phase (due to insulin diffusion through polymer and polymer erosion)[xxv].

Pulmonary delivery: The pulmonary route offers high vascularization, permeability and systemic absorption with respect to thin alveolar epithelium. It has a large surface area of approximately 140 m^2 and lacks mucociliary clearance providing higher insulin residence time. Simultaneously, it has a high proteolytic content, variable absorption profiles that differ from person to person, also requiring a high drug dose[xxvi]. Liposomes, SLNs, Polymeric NPs, nanostructured microparticles and large porous microparticles have been used as novel drug delivery vehicles for pulmonary administration of insulin via oral inhalation technique.

K. P. Amancha et al. (2014) prepared different formulations of microparticles by different layer-by-layer (LbL) nanoassembly of insulin coated by cationic and anionic polyelectrolytes (alternate layers of PDDA and PSS) and administered i.p. to diabetic rats. They found the C_{max} of insulin in serum to be 1345 ± 74.8 μU/mL and 297 ± 43.2 μU/mL with a T_{max} of 0.44 ±0.08 h and 0.94 ± 0.10 h for free insulin solution and 6-LbL-insulin after i.p. administration, respectively. This showed that insulin levels in serum rose rapidly with a sharp decline, whereas, insulin release from carrier was more sustained. Also, the 6-LbL formulation was chosen among 1-,2-,4-,6-,8- and 16-LbL formulations as it had the highest hypoglycemic effect, from 407 ± 46 mg/dL to 8 ± 6 mg/dL serum glucose in 8 hours[xxvii].

Ai-Zheng Chen et al. (2015) loaded poly-L-lactide microspheres with insulin and used ammonium bicarbonate to increase their porosity for i.p. delivery. The hypoglycemic activity of raw insulin was 52.8% and 47.3% for insulin with carrier, at 1 hour after i.p. admistration to mice, showing that the chosen carrier had a mild effect or no effect on i.p. insulin administration[xxviii].

Jie Liu et al. (2008) showed that nebulization of insulin from SLNs increased plasma insulin level from 20 IU/kg to 170 IU/kg and for physical mixture of insulin in PBS and blank SLNs from 20 IU/kg to 68 IU/kg in 4 hours after i.p. admistration to rats, showing the excellent hypoglycemic effect of insulin encapsulated within SLNs[xxix].

S. Al-Qadi et al. (2012) loaded chitosan NPs (of different molecular weights: 113 and 213) with insulin and in turn, encapsulated them in microparticles to study pharmacodynamic effects after intratracheal administration to rats. Both insulin-chitosan NP formulations showed similar and significant hypoglycemic effect decreasing plasma glucose levels by approximately 68% in 1 hour as compared to blank NPs, which showed no hypoglycemic effects[xxx].

Sumio Chono et al. (2009) delivered aerolized liposomes (with dipalmitoyl phosphatidylcholine (DPPC)) containing insulin to rats by i.p. route. The *in vivo* studies showed that in plasma glucose level reduced to 66% and 92% of initial levels in 1 hour, from insulin-DPPC-liposomes and free insulin solution, respectively. On *in vitro* permeation through Calu-3 cell monolayers, plasma glucose level reduced to 70% and 77% of initial levels in 1 hour, from insulin-DPPC-liposomes and free insulin solution, respectively[xxxi].

Kai Shi et al. (2015) fabricated novel spherical NPs from supramolecular self-assembly of insulin, followed by functionalization of insulin by a cationic peptide, ε-poly-L-lysine (EPL). They reported that C_{max} of insulin in serum was 40 mIU/L and 52 mIU/L at a T_{max} of 0.5 h and 2 h after intratracheal administration of free insulin and insulin/EPC/NPs to diabetic rats, respectively. The insulin level gradually declined for insulin/EPC/NPs while abruptly for free insulin over 8 h, showing that insulin, if used along with the above carrier could have prolonged and pronounced hypoglycemic effects[xxxii].

Transdermal delivery: Being a non-invasive drug delivery route, avoiding GI tract and hepatic first-pass effect, the skin unfortunately, has some potential barriers like low permeability of hydrophilic molecules like insulin through lipidic layer of stratum cornuem (ideal for lipophilic molecules of <500 g/mol) . The delivery becomes easier after crossing this toughest layer of highly compact and organized keratinocytes. However, some physical techniques can be applied to temporarily increase stratum corneum permeability to macromolecules like insulin and the delivery can be terminated on removal of the drug delivery system but care should be taken that insulin should not be denatured. Lately, physical techniques like iontoporesis, sonoporesis, electroporation and microneedles have been used[xxxiii].

S.R. Sershen et al. (2002) developed composites of thermally-sensitive N-isopropylacrylamide (NIPAAm) and acrylamide (AAm) hydrogels and optically-active gold-gold sulfide nanoshells for transdermal photothermally modulated drug delivery and showed that the composites could deliver controlled pulsatile doses of insulin in response to near-IR irradiation (800-1200 nm) without any harm to insulin activity. Total insulin release from irradiated and non-irradiated nanoshells at 40 minutes was 28 mg/g d.w. and 13mg/g d.w., respectively[xxxiv].

Seungjun Lee et al. (2002) used cymbal array transducers (37 x 37 x 7 mm^3, <22 g) to demonstrate ultrasound (US) mediated transdermal insulin (ins) delivery *in vivo* on rat models with average glucose levels of 419.1 ± 31.4 mg/dL. For control 1 (ins, no US) and control 2 (saline, US), the glucose level varied no greater than 39.5 ± 59.8 g/dL over a 90 minutes period, indicating insulin alone couldn't alter glucose levels (control 1). For the third group (ins, US 60 min), the glucose level decreased to -75.2 ± 63.2 mg/dL in 30 minutes and -267.5 ± 61.9 mg/dL in 60 minutes. After disabling ultrasound at 60 minutes, the glucose level continued to decrease to -296.7 ± 52.8 mg/dL at 90 minutes. The fourth group (ins, US 20 mins) gave similar results as the third group, with a decrease in blood glucose of -249.3 ± 22.3 mg/dL at 60 minutes, indicating that the time of ultrasound exposure did not matter[xxxv].

More recently, Ming-Hung et al. (2013) used microneedles (composed of starch and gelatin), which dissolved after introduction to skin whitin 5 min, releasing insulin. *In vitro* and *in vivo* histological analysis showed that the microneedles penetrated a depth of 200 μm and 200-250 μm when inserted in porcine skin and rat skin, respectively. The *in vitro* cumulative insulin release profile varied linearly with time till 4 mins, where insulin release was 100%, followed by a constant release profile till 6 mins, showing that the majority of insulin was released within 4 minutes[xxxvi].

CONCLUSION

Among peptide and protein delivery, insulin delivery was discussed in detail highlighting the disadvantages of the conventional s.c. insulin administration like painful expensive injections with loss of fat around injection site and risk of infections. Owing to this, there's a need to exploit other routes of insulin administration utilizing various novel carriers like polymeric NPs, nanoshells, nanospheres, SLNs, liposomes, with some modifications like surface functionalization with appropriate peptide ligands or polymers to enhance absorption or achieve drug targeting. A combination of these carriers (like loading drug inside NPs and in turn, encapsulating them within microparticles) has also been done to protect and safeguard the drug, especially protein drugs as their activity completely depends on structural stability and integrity. The various routes like oral, transdermal, pulmonary and buccal were discussed at length, highlighting the major recent works with respect to the delivery routes and the improvement in the pharmacokinetic and pharmacodynamic profiles.

REFERENCES

[i] G. Walsh. Biopharmaceuticals: Biochemistry and Biotechnology. 2nd ed. England: John Wiley & Sons Ltd; 2003.

[ii] Hogvaard L, Frokjaer S, van de Weert M. Pharmaceutical Formulation Development of peptides and proteins. 2nd ed. United States of America: CRC Press Taylor and Francis Group LLC; 2012.

[iii] Morales JO. Films loaded with insulin-coated nanoparticles (ICNP) as potential platforms for peptide buccal delivery. Colloid Surface B 2014; 122: 38–45.

[iv] Lee VH, Robinson JR. Topical ocular drug delivery: Recent developments and future challenges. J Ocul Pharmacol 1986; 2: 67-108.

[v] American Diabetes Association. Standards of medical care in diabetes. Diabetes Care 2013: 36: S11-66.

[vi] Kitabchi AE, Umpierrez GE, Miles JM, Fisher JN. Hyperglycemic crisis in adult patients with diabetes. Diabetes care 2009; 32: 1335-43.

[vii] Korytkowski M. When oral agents fail: practical barriers to starting insulin. Int J Obes Relat Metab Disord 2002; 26: S18–S24.

[viii] Polonsky WH, Fisher L, Guzman S, Villa-Caballero L, Edelman SV. Psychological insulin resistance in patients with type 2 diabetes. Diabetes Care 2005; 28: 2543–2545.

[ix] L. Heinemann, A. Pfutzner, T. Heise. Alternative routes of administration as an approach to improve insulin therapy: update on dermal, oral, nasal and pulmonary insulin delivery. Curr Pharm Des 2001; 7: 1327-51.

[x] Saffran M, Pansky B, Budd GC, Williams FE. Insulin and the gastrointestinal tract. J Control Release 1997; 46: 89-98.

[xi] Fonte P, Araujo F, Silva C, Pereira C, Reis S, Santos HA et al. Polymer-based nanoparticles for oral insulin delivery: Revisited approaches. Biotechnol Adv 2015; 33: 1342-1354.

[xii] Zhang X, Qi J, Lu Y, He W, Li X, Wu W. Biotinyated liposomes as potential carriers for the oral delivery of insulin, Nanomed Nanotech Biol Med 2014; 10: 167-176.

[xiii] Xiong XY, Li QH, Li YP, Guo L, Li ZL, Gong YC. Pluronic P85/poly(lactic acid) vesicles as novel carrier for oral insulin deliver. Colloid Surface B 2013; 111: 282-288.

[xiv] Li X, Guo S, Zhu C Zhu Q, Gan Y, Rantanen J et al. Intestinal mucosa permeability following insulin delivery using core shell corona nanolipoparticles. Biomaterials 2013; 34: 9678-9687.

[xv] Mukopadhyay P, Chakroborty S, Bhattacharya S, Misra R, Kundu PP. pH-sensitive chitosan/alginate core-shell nanoparticles for efficient and safe oral insulin delivery. Int J Biol Macromol 2015; 71: 640-648.

[xvi] Cho HJ, Oh J, Choo MK, Ha JI, Park Y, Maeng HJ. Chondroitin sulfate-capped gold nanoparticles for the oral delivery of insulin. Int J Biol Macromol 2014; 63: 15-20.

[xvii] Yu F, Li Y, Liu CS, Chen Q, Wang GH, Guo W et al. Enteric-coated capsules filled with mono-disperse micro-particles containing PLGA-lipid-PEG nanoparticles for oral delivery of insulin. Int J Pharm 2015; 484: 181–191.

[xviii] Puratchikody A, Prashanth VV, Mathew VV, Balaram AK. Buccal Drug Delivery: Past, Present and Future - A Review. International Journal of Drug Delivery 2011; 3: 171-184.

[xix] Pathan SA, Iqbal Z, Sahani JK, Talegoankar S, Khar RK, Ahmad FJ. Buccoadhesive drug delivery systems-extensive review on recent patents, Recent Pat Drug Deliv Formul 2008; 2: 177-188.

[xx] HaoJ, Heng PW. Buccal Delivery Systems. Drug Dev Ind Pham 2003; 29: 821-832.

[xxi] Bernstein G. Buccal delivery of insulin: the time is now. Drug Develop Res 2006; 67: 597-609.

[xxii] Senel S, Hincal AA. Drug permeation enhancement via buccal route: possibilities and limitations. J ControlRelease 2001; 72: 133-144.

[xxiii] Owens DR. New horizons-alternative routes for insulin therapy. Nat Rev Drug Discov 2002; 1: 529-540.

[xxiv] Morales JO, Huang S, Williams III RO, McConville JT. Films loaded with insulin-coated nanoparticles (ICNP) as potential platforms for peptide buccal delivery. Colloid Surface B 2014; 122: 38–45.

[xxv] Giovino C, Ayensu I, Tetteh J, Boateng JS. Development and characterization of chitosan films impregnated with insulin loaded PEG-b-PLA NPs: A potential approach for buccal delivery of macromolecules. Int J Pharm 2012; 428: 143-151.

[xxvi] Mandal TK. Inhaled insulin for diabetes mellitus. Am Journal Health-Syst Ph 2005; 62: 1359-1364.

[xxvii] Amancha KP, Balkundi S, Lvov Y, Hussain A. Pulmonary sustained release of insulin from microparticles composed of polyelectrolyte layer-by-layer assembly. Int J Pharm 2014; 466: 96-108.

[xxviii] Chen AZ, Teng N, Wang SB, Kang YQ, Song HF et al. Insulin-loaded poly-L-lactide porous microspheres prepared in supercritical CO_2 for pulmonary drug delivery. J Supercrit Fluids 2015; 101: 117-123.

[xxix] Liu J, Gong T, Fu H, Wang C, Wang X, Chen Q et al. Solid lipid nanoparticles for pulmonary delivery of insulin. Int J Pharm 2008; 356: 333-344.

[xxx] Al-Qadi S, Grenha A, Carrion-Recio D, Seijo B, Remunan-Lopez C. Microencapsulated chitosan nanoparticles for pulmonary protein delivery: in vivo evaluation of insulin-loaded formulations. J Control Release 2012; 157: 383-390.

[xxxi] Chono S, Fukuchi R, Seki T, Morimoto K. Aerosolized liposomes with dipalmitoyl phosphatidylcholine enhance pulmonary insulin delivery. J Control Release 2009; 137: 104-109.

[xxxii] Shi K, Liu Y, Ke L, Fang Y, Yang R, Cui F. Epsilon-poly-L-lysine guided improving pulmonary delivery of supramolecular self-assembled insulin nanospheres. Int J Biol Macromol 2015; 72: 1441-1450.

[xxxiii] Owens DR, Zinman B, Bolli G. Alternative routes of insulin delivery. Diabet Med 2003; 20: 886-896.

[xxxiv] Pulsatile Release of Insulin via Photothermally Modulated Drug Delivery. Texas: Rice University; 2002. Proceedings of the Second Joint EMBS/BMES Conference Sershen SR, Halas NJ, West JL.

[xxxv] Smith NB, Lee S, Shung KK. Ultrasound-mediated transdermal *in vivo* transport of insulin with low profile cymbal arrays. Ultrasound Med Biol 2003; 29: 1205-1210.

[xxxvi] Ling MH, Chen MC. Dissolving polymer microneedle patches for rapid and efficient transdermal delivery of insulin to diabetic rats. Acta Biomater 2013; 9: 8952-8961.

YOUR KNOWLEDGE HAS VALUE

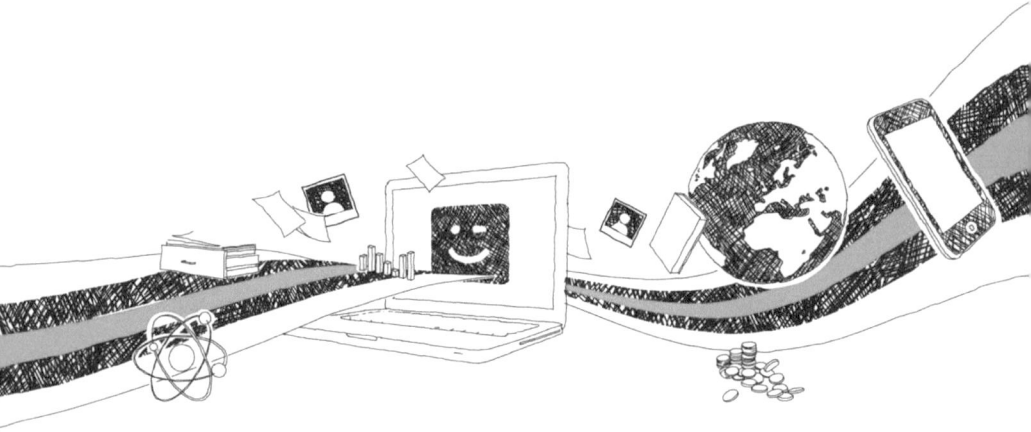

- We will publish your bachelor's and master's thesis, essays and papers

- Your own eBook and book - sold worldwide in all relevant shops

- Earn money with each sale

Upload your text at www.GRIN.com
and publish for free

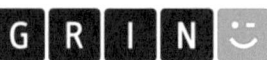